KIDNEY DISEASE
COOKBOOK FOR STAGE 3

The Nephrologist Approved Low Sodium, Low Potassium, Low Phosphorus Recipes to Manage Stage 3 Renal Disease with a 28-Day Meal Plan

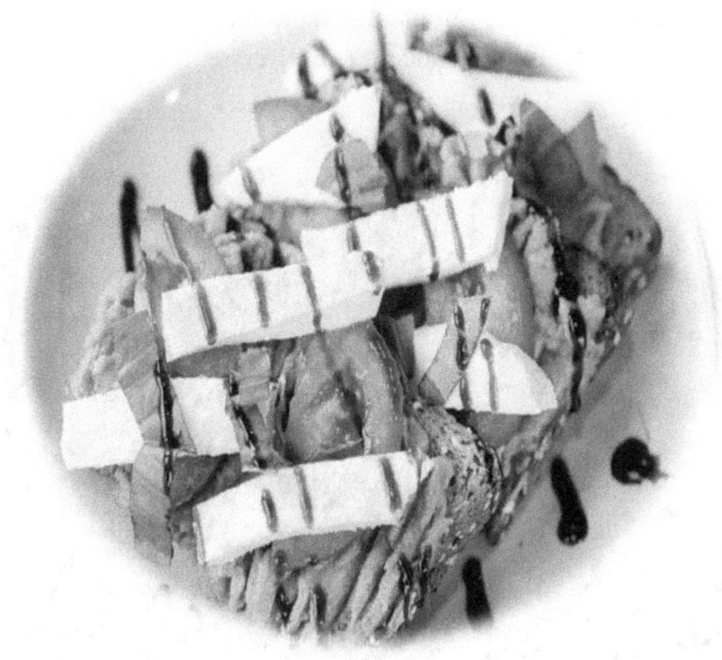

TAYDEN S. WILLIAM

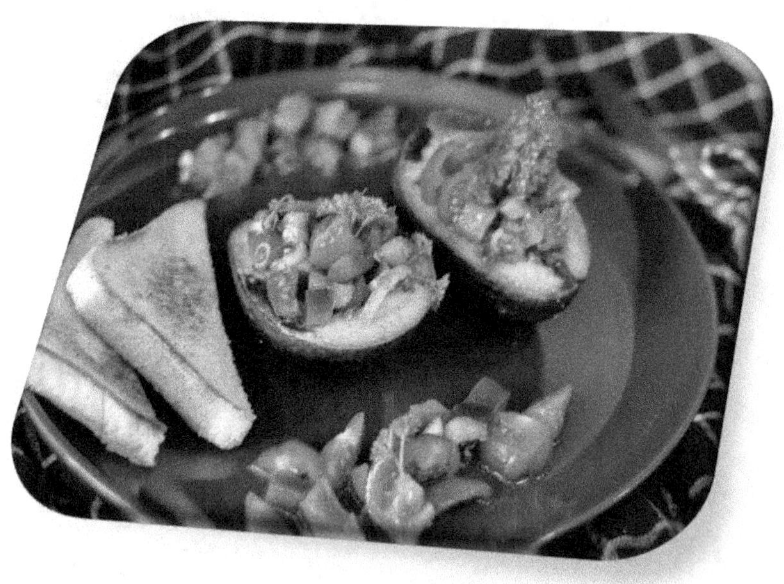

TABLE OF CONTENTS

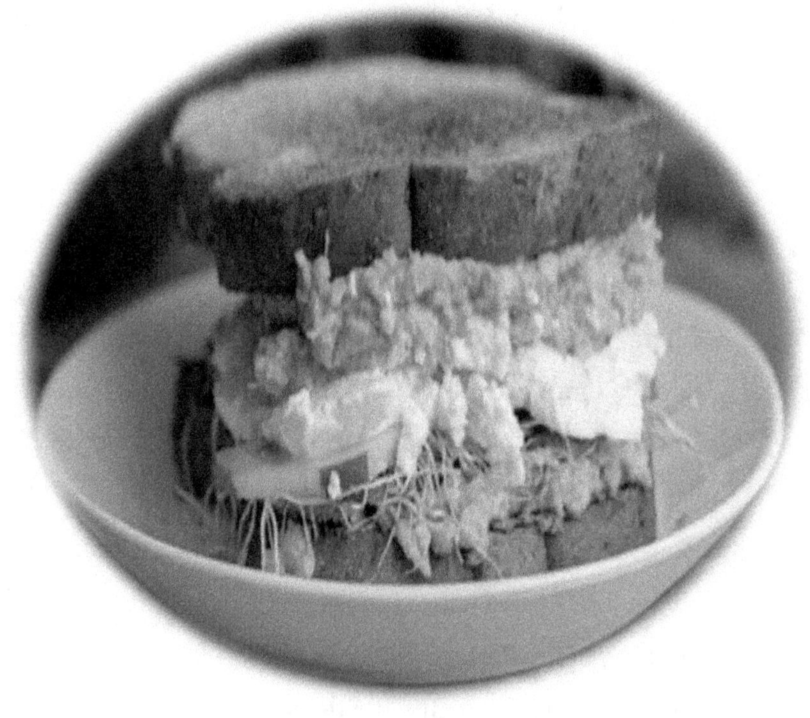

INTRODUCTION

Margaret, a beautiful woman and dear friend from Crestwood, fought the odds, inspiring everyone around her as she embraced life with a vigor that appeared to defy the limits of Stage 3 Kidney Disease. Margaret's tale exemplifies nutrition's transformative potential, serving as a light of hope for those seeking health, life, and happiness.

Margaret's journey began with a diagnosis that could have easily consumed her spirit. Instead, equipped with determination and knowledge, she set out on a gastronomic adventure that would become the foundation of her thriving existence. Her secret? A strict adherence to the recipes in the 'Kidney Disease Cookbook for Stage 3,' which is a collection of nutritional and delectable foods authorized by nephrologists and specifically developed for persons dealing with Stage 3 Renal Disease.

Margaret's story is especially meaningful to me because she is a friend. Witnessing her victory against adversity has provided inspiration and motivation. Her fortitude and determination to adopt a kidney-friendly lifestyle have not only improved her physical health, but have also served as a beacon of hope for countless others suffering similar issues.

Margaret relished the pleasure of tasting tasty meals meticulously prepared to fulfill the demanding needs of her kidney health. As the aroma of kidney-friendly dishes wafted through her kitchen, Margaret realized she could manage her illness without giving up her enjoyment of dining. Her experience demonstrates the efficacy of the recipes in this book.

Tayden S. William, a licensed nutritionist, author, and health coach, is the driving force behind Margaret's success. His path into the realm of wellness stemmed from a desire to assist people reach their health goals. Tayden, the author of this thorough guide, discusses his personal journey from curiosity to professional knowledge in nutrition and holistic health.

Tayden's narrative is one of progression, starting with a basic fascination with the complex dance of food and health. Early on, he realized the enormous impact that a well-balanced diet may have on one's entire health. To fuel his interest, he dived into the field of nutritional research, determined to grasp the complex relationship between specific food choices and the complicated dance that occurs within the human body.

Tayden's constant pursuit of information led him to formal study, where he earned qualifications as a nutritionist and health coach. His voracious curiosity drove him to investigate the complexities of holistic wellness, bringing a thorough awareness of the body-mind relationship into his work. After years of committed research and practical application, Tayden emerged as a beacon of expertise, ready to illuminate the path to healthier life for those suffering from kidney disease.

Tayden's persistent drive to making a positive difference in the lives of people living with Stage 3 Kidney Disease inspired the creation of this book. As the author, he understands the complex relationship between nutrition and renal health, and he is determined to share this information with others to help them on their transformational journeys.

Tayden's intention is to provide readers with not only a collection of meticulously crafted, Nephrologist Approved recipes, but also the knowledge and understanding required to make informed dietary choices. The goal of this book is clear and resolute: to provide a beacon of guidance for individuals navigating the nuances of Stage 3 Renal Disease. This book is more than just a collection of recipes; it's a guide to a healthier, more fulfilled existence.

In the enormous landscape of healthcare, Tayden underlines the critical role of nutrition in kidney disease management. Kidney health is inextricably related to the food we eat, and Tayden's approach is based on the premise that a well-planned diet may be an effective ally in overcoming the challenges faced by Stage 3 Kidney Disease. As the saying goes, "Let food be thy medicine," and this book exemplifies the therapeutic power of conscious, nutritious eating habits.

The following pages are more than just a collection of recipes; they are a comprehensive guide that extends beyond the culinary realm. Tayden invites you on a journey that connects nutrition, well-being, and the delight of experiencing each moment of life. As you turn the pages of the 'Kidney Disease Cookbook for Stage 3,' imagine a path lighted by Margaret's triumphs, guided by Tayden's expertise, and enriched by the knowledge that food is more than simply nourishment; it is a powerful instrument for healing and flourishing.

CHAPTER ONE

Understanding Stage 3 Kidney Disease

In the maze of kidney health, Stage 3 Renal Disease is a watershed moment where understanding, action, and dietary adjustments can drastically affect the course of one's well-being. This chapter looks into the complex landscape of Stage 3 Renal Disease, exploring its ramifications and emphasizing the importance of a specific diet, notably one low in sodium, potassium, and phosphorus.

Stage 3 Renal Disease, often known as moderate kidney impairment, is a significant point in the evolution of renal dysfunction. At this point, the kidneys' ability to filter waste from the blood is hampered. Individuals may be asymptomatic, making the disease a stealthy and insidious force that quietly undermines health while displaying few symptoms.

The ramifications of Stage 3 Renal Disease go beyond the kidney's basic functions. It is a prelude to more severe stages, and appropriate therapy during this period is critical for delaying development and preserving kidney function. Understanding the significance of this stage is the foundation for the journey described in this book.

Why Dietary Changes Matter

Dietary modifications take center stage in the management Stage 3 Renal Disease. The kidneys, which regulate the body's fluid and electrolyte balance, become especially sensitive to the composition of the foods we eat. As the kidneys struggle to filter waste efficiently, the buildup of certain compounds, such as salt, potassium, and phosphorus, can exacerbate the organs' problems.

Sodium:

Sodium, a common component of our everyday diet, has an important but frequently overlooked role in kidney health. The importance of following a low-sodium diet in Stage 3 Renal Disease cannot be emphasized. The tendency of sodium to hold water can result in fluid retention, which raises blood pressure and puts additional strain on impaired kidneys.

As people move through Stage 3 Renal Disease, maintaining blood pressure becomes an important part of overall therapy. A low-sodium diet not only helps to control blood pressure, but it also reduces the danger of fluid overload, relieving the burden on the kidneys and fostering a healthier fluid balance in the body.

Potassium:

Potassium, an essential mineral for nerve and muscle function, must be carefully monitored in the setting of Stage 3 Renal Disease. Damaged kidneys struggle to control potassium levels, which can lead to major health complications. A low-potassium diet is necessary to avoid hyperkalemia, a disorder marked by increased potassium levels in the blood.

A low-potassium diet consists of eating foods with lower potassium content to avoid overloading the kidneys with the chore of filtering excess potassium from the bloodstream. Individuals with Stage 3 Renal Disease who carefully manage their potassium intake can assist maintain the delicate balance essential for good kidney function.

Phosphorus:

Phosphorus, an essential mineral for bone health, acts as a silent saboteur in the presence of poor renal function. In Stage 3 Renal Disease, the kidneys struggle to remove excess phosphorus, which accumulates in the circulation. Elevated phosphorus levels can contribute to mineral and bone diseases, which harm the skeletal system.

A low-phosphorus diet is critical for reducing the consequences of phosphorus buildup. Individuals with Stage 3 Renal Disease can exert some control over this often overlooked but significant factor to renal dysfunction by eating foods with lower phosphorus content.

The importance of following a low sodium, low potassium, and low phosphorus diet resides not only in individual limits, but also in the overall synergy of these dietary adjustments. Individuals with Stage 3 Renal Disease can achieve the delicate balance necessary for good kidney function by adopting a complete nutritional approach.

The complex dance of sodium, potassium, and phosphorus within the body needs an informed and deliberate approach to dietary selection. Recognizing the interdependence of these aspects enables people to adopt dietary choices that promote renal function, lower the risk of problems, and improve overall health.

As we embark on this trip through the maze of Stage 3 Renal Disease, it is critical that we grasp the complex relationship between our dietary habits and kidney health. This chapter serves as a foundation, outlining the problems presented by Stage 3 Renal Disease and emphasizing the critical role that a low sodium, low potassium, and low phosphorus diet can play in treating and, in some cases, preventing the course of this condition.

Shopping List

Proteins:

- Chicken breasts
- Salmon fillets
- Tofu
- Shrimp
- Cod fillets
- Lentils

Dairy:

- Low-sodium Greek yogurt
- Low-sodium cottage cheese
- Low-potassium almond milk

- Low-sodium coconut water

Fruits:
- Berries (strawberries, blueberries, raspberries)
- Banana
- Kiwi
- Mango
- Pineapple
- Pear
- Orange
- Apple
- Papaya
- Cherries

Vegetables:
- Spinach
- Cucumber
- Mint
- Avocado
- Blueberries
- Broccoli
- Asparagus
- Eggplant
- Tomato
- Cauliflower
- Sweet potatoes

Grains and Carbohydrates:

- Quinoa
- Brown rice
- Whole wheat roll
- Basmati rice

Nuts and Seeds:

- Almonds
- Walnuts
- Pumpkin seeds
- Sesame seeds

Legumes:

- Chickpeas
- Edamame
- Lentils

Herbs and Spices:

- Garlic powder
- Cumin
- Paprika
- Fresh ginger
- Fresh herbs (e.g., basil, parsley)

Condiments and Sauces:

- Low-sodium soy sauce
- Olive oil (low sodium)
- Low-phosphorus almond butter

- Hummus (low sodium)

Baking and Cooking Essentials:
- Nutritional yeast
- Sea salt

Sweeteners:
- Honey

Dried Fruits:
- Unsweetened dried cranberries

Extras:
- Low-sodium rice cakes

Frozen Foods:
- Frozen mixed berries

Miscellaneous:
- Chia seeds

Ensure to check the labels for sodium, potassium, and phosphorus content in packaged items. Adjust quantities based on the number of servings you plan to prepare.

CHAPTER TWO

Breakfast Recipes

Quinoa Breakfast Bowl

Prep Time: 10 minutes
Cooking Time: 15 minutes
Ingredients:

- 1/2 cup quinoa, rinsed
- 1 cup almond milk (low potassium)
- 1/2 cup blueberries
- 1 tablespoon chopped almonds (low phosphorus)
- 1 teaspoon honey (optional)

Method:

1. In a saucepan, combine the quinoa and the almond milk.
2. Bring to a boil, then reduce to a simmer to cook the quinoa.
3. Top with blueberries, sliced almonds, and honey, if desired.

Nutritional Info:

Calories: 300 / Protein: 8g / Fiber: 5g / Potassium: 150mg / Phosphorus: 80mg / Sodium: 50mg

Egg White Veggie Omelette

Prep Time: 5 minutes
Cooking Time: 10 minutes
Ingredients:

- 3 egg whites
- 1/4 cup diced bell peppers
- 1/4 cup diced zucchini
- 1 tablespoon olive oil (low sodium)
- Salt and pepper to taste

Method:

1. In a mixing basin, whisk together the egg whites.
2. Sauté the bell peppers and zucchini in olive oil until soft.
3. Pour egg whites over vegetables, heat until set, then fold.

Nutritional Info:
Calories: 120 / Protein: 15g / Fiber: 2g / Potassium: 200mg / Phosphorus: 100mg / Sodium: 80mg

Greek Yogurt Parfait

Prep Time: 5 minutes
Cooking Time: 0 minutes
Ingredients:

- 1/2 cup low-fat Greek yogurt
- 1/4 cup strawberries, sliced
- 1 tablespoon chia seeds

- 1 tablespoon chopped walnuts (low phosphorus)
- Drizzle of honey (optional)

Method:
1. In a glass, combine yogurt, strawberries, chia seeds, and chopped walnuts.
2. Drizzle with honey if preferred.

Nutritional Info:
Calories: 200 / Protein: 12g / Fiber: 4g / Potassium: 180mg / Phosphorus: 70mg / Sodium: 60mg

Buckwheat Pancakes

Prep Time: 15 minutes
Cooking Time: 10 minutes
Ingredients:
- 1/2 cup buckwheat flour
- 1/2 cup almond milk (low potassium)
- 1/2 teaspoon baking powder
- 1 tablespoon applesauce (low potassium)
- Fresh berries for topping

Method:
1. Mix together buckwheat flour, almond milk, baking powder, and applesauce.
2. Cook spoonful of batter on the griddle until bubbles appear, then flip.

Calories: 180 / Protein: 6g / Fiber: 4g / Potassium: 120mg / Phosphorus: 60mg / Sodium: 40mg

Chia Seed Pudding

Prep Time: 5 minutes
Cooking Time: 0 minutes (overnight refrigeration)
Ingredients:

- 2 tablespoons chia seeds
- 1/2 cup almond milk (low potassium)
- 1/4 teaspoon vanilla extract
- Sliced kiwi for topping

Method:

1. Combine chia seeds, almond milk, and vanilla essence.
2. Refrigerate overnight, then top with sliced kiwi to serve.

Nutritional Info:

Calories: 120 / Protein: 4g / Fiber: 8g / Potassium: 90mg / Phosphorus: 50mg / Sodium: 20mg

Sweet Potato Hash Browns

Prep Time: 15 minutes
Cooking Time: 20 minutes
Ingredients:

- 1 medium sweet potato, grated

- 1 tablespoon olive oil (low sodium)
- 1/4 teaspoon garlic powder
- Fresh parsley for garnish

Method:
1. Squeeze the moisture from the grated sweet potato.
2. Sauté garlic powder with olive oil until golden brown.

Nutritional Info:
Calories: 150 / Protein: 2g / Fiber: 4g / Potassium: 180mg / Phosphorus: 60mg / Sodium: 30mg

Oatmeal with Berries and Almond Butter

Prep Time: 5 minutes
Cooking Time: 5 minutes
Ingredients:
- 1/2 cup old-fashioned oats
- 1 cup water
- 1/4 cup mixed berries
- 1 tablespoon almond butter (low phosphorus)

Method:
1. Cook the oats in water until they reach your preferred consistency.
2. Garnish with mixed berries and a dab of almond butter.

Nutritional Info:

Calories: 250 / Protein: 7g / Fiber: 6g / Potassium: 120mg / Phosphorus: 70mg / Sodium: 10mg

Cottage Cheese and Pineapple Bowl

Prep Time: 5 minutes
Cooking Time: 0 minutes
Ingredients:

- 1/2 cup low-fat cottage cheese
- 1/2 cup fresh pineapple, diced
- 1 tablespoon pumpkin seeds (low phosphorus)

Method:

1. In a mixing dish, combine the cottage cheese and the cubed pineapple.
2. Sprinkle with pumpkin seeds.

Nutritional Info:

Calories: 180 / Protein: 15g / Fiber: 2g / Potassium: 180mg / Phosphorus: 50mg / Sodium: 90mg

Avocado Toast with Tomato and Basil

Prep Time: 5 minutes
Cooking Time: 0 minutes
Ingredients:

- 1 slice whole grain bread
- 1/2 ripe avocado, mashed
- 1/2 tomato, sliced

- Fresh basil leaves for garnish

Method:
1. Toast the bread.
2. Spread mashed avocado on the toast, then top with chopped tomatoes and basil.

Nutritional Info:
Calories: 200 / Protein: 5g / Fiber: 7g / Potassium: 250mg / Phosphorus: 80mg / Sodium: 120mg

Rice Cake with Smoked Salmon

Prep Time: 5 minutes
Cooking Time: 0 minutes
Ingredients:
- 1 rice cake
- 2 ounces smoked salmon
- 1 tablespoon cream cheese (low phosphorus)
- Fresh dill for garnish

Method:
1. Spread cream cheese over the rice cake.
2. Add smoked salmon and garnish with fresh dill.

Nutritional Info:
Calories: 180 / Protein: 12g / Fiber: 1g / Potassium: 200mg / Phosphorus: 60mg / Sodium: 200mg

Lunch Recipes

Grilled Lemon Herb Chicken Salad

Prep Time: 15 minutes
Cooking Time: 15 minutes
Ingredients:

- 4 ounces boneless, skinless chicken breast
- Mixed greens
- Cherry tomatoes, halved
- Cucumber, sliced
- Olive oil (low sodium)
- Lemon juice
- Fresh herbs (rosemary, thyme)
- Salt and pepper to taste

Method:

1. Season the chicken with herbs, salt, and pepper.
2. Grill until cooked through, then slice.
3. Make a salad with mixed greens, tomatoes, and cucumber.
4. Drizzle with olive oil and lemon juice, then top with grilled chicken.

Nutritional Info:

Calories: 300 / Protein: 25g / Fiber: 4g / Potassium: 300mg / Phosphorus: 150mg / Sodium: 100mg

Vegetarian Quinoa Stuffed Bell Peppers

Prep Time: 20 minutes
Cooking Time: 30 minutes
Ingredients:

- 1/2 cup quinoa, cooked
- Bell peppers, halved
- Black beans, drained and rinsed (low phosphorus)
- Corn kernels
- Diced tomatoes
- Cumin, paprika, salt, and pepper to taste

Method:

1. Combine cooked quinoa with black beans, corn, and sliced tomatoes.
2. Season with cumin, paprika, salt, and pepper.
3. Stuff the mixture into halved bell peppers and bake until cooked.

Nutritional Info:
Calories: 250 / Protein: 10g / Fiber: 8g / Potassium: 200mg / Phosphorus: 100mg / Sodium: 80mg

Salmon and Asparagus Foil Pack

Prep Time: 10 minutes
Cooking Time: 20 minutes
Ingredients:

- 4 ounces salmon fillet
- Asparagus spears

- Lemon slices
- Olive oil (low sodium)
- Dill, salt, and pepper to taste

Method:
1. Place the salmon on a piece of foil, surrounded by asparagus.
2. Drizzle with olive oil, then add lemon slices and season with dill, salt, and pepper.
3. Seal the foil and bake until the salmon is cooked through.

Nutritional Info:
Calories: 280 / Protein: 25g / Fiber: 3g / Potassium: 300mg / Phosphorus: 200mg / Sodium: 60mg

Eggplant and Tomato Bake

Prep Time: 15 minutes
Cooking Time: 25 minutes
Ingredients:
- 1 medium eggplant, sliced
- Roma tomatoes, sliced
- Olive oil (low sodium)
- Garlic, minced
- Basil, oregano, salt, and pepper to taste
- Grated mozzarella cheese (optional)

Method:

1. Layer eggplant and tomato slices in a baking dish.
2. Drizzle with olive oil and season with minced garlic, herbs, salt, and pepper.
3. Bake until the vegetables are soft.
4. Optional: Sprinkle with grated mozzarella cheese and broil until it melts.

Nutritional Info:

Calories: 220 / Protein: 5g / Fiber: 8g / Potassium: 250mg / Phosphorus: 100mg / Sodium: 40mg

Lentil and Vegetable Soup

Prep Time: 10 minutes
Cooking Time: 30 minutes
Ingredients:

- 1/2 cup dry lentils, rinsed
- Carrots, chopped
- Celery, chopped
- Onion, diced
- Low-sodium vegetable broth
- Bay leaves, thyme, salt, and pepper to taste

Method:

1. Put lentils, carrots, celery, and onion in a saucepan.
2. Combine the vegetable broth, bay leaves, thyme, salt, and pepper.
3. Simmer until the lentils and veggies are soft.

Nutritional Info:

Calories: 180 / Protein: 12g / Fiber: 8g / Potassium: 300mg / Phosphorus: 150mg / Sodium: 60mg

Shrimp and Spinach Salad

Prep Time: 10 minutes
Cooking Time: 5 minutes
Ingredients:

- 4 ounces shrimp, peeled and deveined
- Fresh spinach leaves
- Cherry tomatoes, halved
- Avocado, diced
- Olive oil (low sodium)
- Balsamic vinegar
- Salt and pepper to taste

Method:

1. Sauté the shrimp until done.
2. Combine the spinach, tomatoes, and avocado in a bowl.
3. Garnish with cooked shrimp and drizzle with olive oil and balsamic vinegar.

Nutritional Info:

Calories: 220 / Protein: 20g / Fiber: 6g / Potassium: 250mg / Phosphorus: 180mg / Sodium: 80mg

Chicken and Vegetable Stir-Fry

Prep Time: 15 minutes
Cooking Time: 15 minutes
Ingredients:
- 4 ounces boneless, skinless chicken breast, sliced
- Broccoli florets
- Bell peppers, sliced
- Snap peas
- Low-sodium soy sauce
- Ginger, minced
- Garlic, minced
- Brown rice (optional, cooked separately)

Method:
1. Stir-fry the chicken until done and set aside.
2. Stir-fry the vegetables with ginger and garlic.
3. Stir in cooked chicken and soy sauce until well heated.
4. Serve with brown rice if preferred.

Nutritional Info:
Calories: 280 / Protein: 25g / Fiber: 6g / Potassium: 300mg / Phosphorus: 150mg / Sodium: 120mg

Turkey and Vegetable Wrap

Prep Time: 10 minutes
Cooking Time: 10 minutes
Ingredients:

- 4 ounces ground turkey
- Whole grain wrap
- Lettuce leaves
- Tomato, sliced
- Cucumber, sliced
- Mustard (low sodium)
- Hummus (low phosphorus)

Method:

1. Cook the ground turkey until browned.
2. Spread hummus on the wrap, then add lettuce, turkey, tomato, and cucumber.
3. Drizzle with mustard, wrap and serve.

Nutritional Info:
Calories: 320 / Protein: 20g / Fiber: 8g / Potassium: 200mg / Phosphorus: 100mg / Sodium: 80mg

Mushroom and Spinach Frittata

Prep Time: 10 minutes
Cooking Time: 20 minutes
Ingredients:

- 3 eggs, beaten
- Mushrooms, sliced

- Fresh spinach leaves
- Onion, diced
- Low-fat feta cheese
- Olive oil (low sodium)
- Salt and pepper to taste

Method:
1. Sauté the mushrooms and onions in olive oil until tender.
2. Add the spinach and simmer until wilted.
3. Pour beaten eggs over the vegetables, top with feta, and simmer until set.

Nutritional Info:
Calories: 250 / Protein: 18g / Fiber: 4g / Potassium: 250mg / Phosphorus: 120mg / Sodium: 90mg

Tuna and White Bean Salad

Prep Time: 10 minutes
Cooking Time: 0 minutes
Ingredients:
- 1 can (5 ounces) tuna, drained
- White beans, rinsed and drained
- Cherry tomatoes, halved
- Red onion, finely chopped
- Olive oil (low sodium)
- Lemon juice
- Fresh parsley, chopped

- Salt and pepper to taste

Method:
1. Sauté the mushrooms and onions in olive oil until tender.
2. Add the spinach and simmer until wilted.
3. Pour beaten eggs over the vegetables, top with feta, and simmer until set.

Nutritional Info:
Calories: 290 / Protein: 25g / Fiber: 8g / Potassium: 350mg / Phosphorus: 200mg / Sodium: 120mg

Dinner Recipes
Baked Lemon Herb Cod
Prep Time: 10 minutes
Cooking Time: 20 minutes
Ingredients:
- 6 ounces cod fillet
- Lemon juice
- Fresh herbs (dill, parsley)
- Olive oil (low sodium)
- Garlic powder
- Salt and pepper to taste

Method:
1. Place the cod on a baking pan and season with lemon juice and olive oil.

2. Season with fresh herbs, garlic powder, salt, and pepper.
3. Bake until the fish flaked easily.

Nutritional Info:

Calories: 200 / Protein: 25g / Fiber: 2g / Potassium: 250mg / Phosphorus: 150mg / Sodium: 80mg

Vegetable and Chickpea Curry

Prep Time: 15 minutes
Cooking Time: 25 minutes
Ingredients:

- 1 can (15 ounces) chickpeas, drained
- Mixed vegetables (zucchini, bell peppers, carrots)
- Coconut milk (low phosphorus)
- Curry powder, turmeric, cumin
- Brown rice (optional, cooked separately)

Method:

1. Sauté the mixed vegetables in a pan.
2. Combine chickpeas, coconut milk, and seasonings.
3. Simmer until the vegetables are soft.
4. Serve with brown rice if preferred.

Nutritional Info:

Calories: 300 / Protein: 12g / Fiber: 8g / Potassium: 300mg / Phosphorus: 180mg / Sodium: 70mg

Grilled Chicken and Quinoa Salad

Prep Time: 15 minutes
Cooking Time: 15 minutes
Ingredients:

- 4 ounces grilled chicken breast, sliced
- Quinoa, cooked
- Cherry tomatoes, halved
- Cucumber, diced
- Olive oil (low sodium)
- Balsamic vinegar
- Fresh basil, chopped
- Salt and pepper to taste

Method:

1. Combine grilled chicken, quinoa, tomatoes, and cucumbers.
2. Drizzle with olive oil and balsamic vinegar.
3. Add the chopped basil, salt, and pepper.

Nutritional Info:
Calories: 320 / Protein: 25g / Fiber: 6g / Potassium: 250mg / Phosphorus: 200mg / Sodium: 90mg

Turkey and Vegetable Skewers

Prep Time: 20 minutes
Cooking Time: 15 minutes
Ingredients:

- 4 ounces ground turkey

- Cherry tomatoes
- Bell peppers, cut into chunks
- Red onion, cut into wedges
- Olive oil (low sodium)
- Rosemary, thyme, salt, and pepper to taste

Method:
1. Combine ground turkey, herbs, salt, and pepper.
2. Form into small skewers, alternating with vegetables.
3. Grill until the turkey is done and the vegetables are soft.

Nutritional Info:
Calories: 250 / Protein: 20g / Fiber: 4g / Potassium: 200mg / Phosphorus: 120mg / Sodium: 60mg

Egg Fried Cauliflower Rice

Prep Time: 10 minutes
Cooking Time: 15 minutes
Ingredients:
- Cauliflower, grated
- Eggs, beaten
- Peas
- Carrots, diced
- Low-sodium soy sauce
- Olive oil (low sodium)
- Ginger, minced

- Garlic, minced

Method:
1. Sauté carrots and peas in olive oil with ginger and garlic.
2. Add the grated cauliflower and simmer until tender.
3. Push the vegetables to the side, add the beaten eggs, and scramble.
4. Combine all ingredients, then add soy sauce and mix.

Nutritional Info:
Calories: 180 / Protein: 10g / Fiber: 6g / Potassium: 220mg / Phosphorus: 80mg / Sodium: 50mg

Salmon and Broccoli Bake
Prep Time: 15 minutes
Cooking Time: 20 minutes
Ingredients:
- 6 ounces salmon fillet
- Broccoli florets
- Lemon slices
- Olive oil (low sodium)
- Dill, salt, and pepper to taste

Method:
1. Place salmon on a baking sheet and surround with broccoli.

2. Drizzle with olive oil, then add lemon slices and season with dill, salt, and pepper.
3. Bake until the salmon is cooked through.

Nutritional Info:
Calories: 280 / Protein: 25g / Fiber: 4g / Potassium: 350mg / Phosphorus: 200mg / Sodium: 60mg

Mushroom and Spinach Stuffed Chicken Breast

Prep Time: 20 minutes
Cooking Time: 25 minutes
Ingredients:
- 2 boneless, skinless chicken breasts
- Mushrooms, chopped
- Fresh spinach
- Low-fat feta cheese
- Olive oil (low sodium)
- Garlic, minced
- Salt and pepper to taste

Method:
1. Sauté mushrooms, spinach, and garlic in olive oil.
2. Slice the chicken breasts horizontally and stuff with the mushroom and spinach mixture.
3. Bake until the chicken is done, then sprinkle with feta.

Nutritional Info:

Calories: 320 / Protein: 30g / Fiber: 5g / Potassium: 300mg / Phosphorus: 150mg / Sodium: 80mg

Lentil and Vegetable Casserole

Prep Time: 15 minutes
Cooking Time: 30 minutes
Ingredients:

- 1 cup dry lentils, rinsed
- Mixed vegetables (carrots, celery, peas)
- Low-sodium vegetable broth
- Onion, diced
- Garlic, minced
- Thyme, rosemary, salt, and pepper to taste

Method:

1. Combine lentils, veggies, broth, onion, garlic, and spices in a casserole dish.
2. Bake until the lentils and veggies are soft.

Nutritional Info:

Calories: 280 / Protein: 18g / Fiber: 10g / Potassium: 350mg / Phosphorus: 180mg / Sodium: 70mg

Shrimp and Zucchini Noodles

Prep Time: 15 minutes
Cooking Time: 10 minutes
Ingredients:

- 4 ounces shrimp, peeled and deveined
- Zucchini, spiralized
- Cherry tomatoes, halved
- Olive oil (low sodium)
- Lemon juice
- Garlic, minced
- Fresh basil, chopped
- Salt and pepper to taste

Method:

1. Sauté the shrimp in olive oil with minced garlic.
2. Add the zucchini noodles and simmer until soft.
3. Toss in cherry tomatoes, lemon juice, basil, salt, and pepper.

Nutritional Info:

Calories: 250 / Protein: 20g / Fiber: 5g / Potassium: 300mg / Phosphorus: 150mg / Sodium: 90mg

Tofu and Vegetable Stir-Fry

Prep Time: 15 minutes
Cooking Time: 15 minutes
Ingredients:

- 6 ounces firm tofu, cubed
- Broccoli florets
- Snow peas
- Bell peppers, sliced
- Low-sodium soy sauce
- Sesame oil (low sodium)
- Ginger, minced
- Garlic, minced
- Brown rice (optional, cooked separately)

Method:

1. Sauté the tofu till golden brown.
2. Stir-fry the vegetables with ginger and garlic.
3. Stir in the tofu, soy sauce, and sesame oil until well cooked.
4. Serve with brown rice if preferred.

Nutritional Info:

Calories: 290 / Protein: 18g / Fiber: 8g / Potassium: 250mg / Phosphorus: 120mg / Sodium: 100mg

Dessert Recipes

Chia Seed and Berry Parfait

Prep Time: 10 minutes
Cooking Time: 0 minutes
Ingredients:

- 2 tablespoons chia seeds
- 1/2 cup almond milk (low potassium)
- Mixed berries
- 1 tablespoon chopped almonds (low phosphorus)
- 1 teaspoon honey (optional)

Method:

1. Combine chia seeds and almond milk; refrigerate until pudding-like.
2. Layer chia pudding with mixed berries and sliced almonds.
3. Drizzle with honey if preferred.

Nutritional Info:
Calories: 150 / Protein: 5g / Fiber: 8g / Potassium: 90mg / Phosphorus: 50mg / Sodium: 20mg

Baked Cinnamon Apples

Prep Time: 10 minutes
Cooking Time: 20 minutes
Ingredients:

- 2 apples, sliced
- Cinnamon

- 1 tablespoon chopped walnuts (low phosphorus)
- 1 tablespoon maple syrup (low potassium)

Method:

1. Toss the apple slices with cinnamon and walnuts.
2. Drizzle with maple syrup.
3. Bake until the apples are soft.

Nutritional Info:

Calories: 180 / Protein: 2g / Fiber: 6g / Potassium: 120mg / Phosphorus: 40mg / Sodium: 5mg

Coconut and Mango Sorbet

Prep Time: 15 minutes
Freezing Time: 4 hours
Ingredients:

- 1 cup coconut milk (low potassium)
- 1 cup frozen mango chunks
- 1 tablespoon agave nectar (low phosphorus)

Method:

1. Blend coconut milk with frozen mango until smooth.
2. Sweeten with agave nectar.
3. Freeze until sorbet consistency.

Nutritional Info:

Calories: 220 / Protein: 2g / Fiber: 3g / Potassium: 100mg / Phosphorus: 30mg / Sodium: 10mg

Greek Yogurt with Berries

Prep Time: 5 minutes
Cooking Time: 0 minutes
Ingredients:

- 1/2 cup low-fat Greek yogurt
- Mixed berries
- 1 tablespoon sunflower seeds (low phosphorus)
- 1 teaspoon honey (optional)

Method:

1. Put Greek yogurt in a bowl.
2. Top with a mix of berries and sunflower seeds.
3. Drizzle with honey if preferred.

Nutritional Info:

Calories: 200 / Protein: 12g / Fiber: 4g / Potassium: 180mg / Phosphorus: 50mg / Sodium: 60mg

Peach and Raspberry Popsicles

Prep Time: 10 minutes
Freezing Time: 4 hours
Ingredients:

- 1 cup fresh or frozen peaches
- 1/2 cup raspberries
- 1 cup coconut water (low potassium)
- 1 tablespoon chia seeds

Method:
1. Blend the peaches, raspberries, and coconut water.
2. Stir in the chia seeds.
3. Pour into popsicle molds and freeze.

Nutritional Info:
Calories: 120 / Protein: 2g / Fiber: 6g / Potassium: 150mg /
Phosphorus: 40mg / Sodium: 20mg

Banana and Almond Butter Bites

Prep Time: 5 minutes
Cooking Time: 0 minutes
Ingredients:
- 1 banana, sliced
- Almond butter (low phosphorus)
- 1 tablespoon shredded coconut (low phosphorus)

Method:
1. Spread almond butter over banana slices.
2. Sprinkle with shredded coconut.

Nutritional Info:
Calories: 180 / Protein: 4g / Fiber: 4g / Potassium: 300mg /
Phosphorus: 60mg / Sodium: 10mg

Chocolate Avocado Mousse

Prep Time: 10 minutes
Chilling Time: 2 hours
Ingredients:

- 2 ripe avocados
- 1/4 cup cocoa powder
- 1/4 cup agave nectar (low phosphorus)
- 1 teaspoon vanilla extract

Method:

1. Blend the avocados, cocoa powder, agave nectar, and vanilla until creamy.
2. Chill in the refrigerator for at least two hours.

Nutritional Info:

Calories: 250 / Protein: 4g / Fiber: 10g / Potassium: 350mg / Phosphorus: 80mg / Sodium: 10mg

Rice Pudding with Cinnamon

Prep Time: 5 minutes
Cooking Time: 30 minutes
Ingredients:

- 1/2 cup Arborio rice
- 2 cups almond milk (low potassium)
- Cinnamon
- 1 tablespoon raisins (low phosphorus)

Method:
1. Cook the rice in almond milk until creamy.
2. Sweeten with cinnamon and mix in raisins.

Nutritional Info:
Calories: 220 / Protein: 3g / Fiber: 2g / Potassium: 120mg /
Phosphorus: 40mg / Sodium: 20mg

Walnut and Date Energy Balls

Prep Time: 15 minutes
Chilling Time: 30 minutes
Ingredients:
- 1 cup walnuts (low phosphorus)
- 1 cup dates, pitted
- 1/2 teaspoon vanilla extract
- Shredded coconut for rolling (optional)

Method:
1. Blend the walnuts, dates, and vanilla until a sticky substance forms.
2. Roll into bite-sized balls.
3. *Optional: Roll in shredded coconut and chill.*

Nutritional Info:
Calories: 180 / Protein: 4g / Fiber: 3g / Potassium: 150mg /
Phosphorus: 60mg / Sodium: 5mg

Berry Oat Crumble Bars

Prep Time: 20 minutes
Baking Time: 25 minutes
Ingredients:

- 1 cup oats
- Mixed berries
- 1/4 cup almond flour
- 2 tablespoons coconut oil (low sodium)
- 1 tablespoon maple syrup (low potassium)

Method:

1. Combine the oats, almond flour, melted coconut oil, and maple syrup.
2. Press half of the mixture into a baking dish.
3. Spread the berries on the base, then top with the remaining oat mixture.
4. Bake until golden brown, then cool before cutting into bars.

Nutritional Info:
Calories: 230 / Protein: 5g / Fiber: 6g / Potassium: 100mg / Phosphorus: 30mg / Sodium: 10mg

Smoothie Recipes

Berry Blast Smoothie

Prep Time: 5 minutes
Blending Time: 2 minutes
Ingredients:

- 1/2 cup mixed berries (strawberries, blueberries, raspberries)
- 1/2 banana
- 1/2 cup low-potassium coconut water
- Ice cubes

Method:

1. Blend the berries, banana, and coconut water until smooth.
2. Add ice cubes and blend again until the desired smoothness is achieved.

Nutritional Info:

Calories: 120 / Protein: 2g / Fiber: 6g / Potassium: 150mg / Phosphorus: 40mg / Sodium: 10mg

Cucumber Mint Refresher

Prep Time: 5 minutes
Blending Time: 2 minutes
Ingredients:

- 1/2 cucumber, peeled and sliced
- Handful of fresh mint leaves
- 1/2 cup low-sodium yogurt

- Splash of water
- Ice cubes

Method:

1. Blend the cucumber, mint, yogurt, and water until smooth.
2. To achieve a refreshing texture, add ice cubes and mix.

Nutritional Info:

Calories: 90 / Protein: 4g / Fiber: 2g / Potassium: 120mg / Phosphorus: 60mg / Sodium: 30mg

Pineapple Ginger Zing

Prep Time: 5 minutes
Blending Time: 2 minutes
Ingredients:

- 1/2 cup pineapple chunks
- Small piece of fresh ginger
- 1/2 cup low-potassium coconut water
- Ice cubes

Method:

1. Blend the pineapple, ginger, and coconut water until smooth.
2. Blend in ice cubes to create a delicious tropical flavor.

Nutritional Info:

Calories: 100 / Protein: 1g / Fiber: 2g / Potassium: 100mg / Phosphorus: 30mg / Sodium: 20mg

Avocado Banana Bliss

Prep Time: 5 minutes
Blending Time: 2 minutes
Ingredients:

- 1/2 avocado
- 1/2 banana
- 1 cup low-sodium almond milk
- Ice cubes

Method:

1. Blend the avocado, banana, and almond milk until creamy.
2. Blend with ice cubes for a smooth and delicious delight.

Nutritional Info:

Calories: 180 / Protein: 3g / Fiber: 6g / Potassium: 220mg / Phosphorus: 50mg / Sodium: 80mg

Strawberry Kiwi Delight

Prep Time: 5 minutes
Blending Time: 2 minutes
Ingredients:

- 1/2 cup strawberries
- 1 kiwi, peeled and sliced
- 1/2 cup low-sodium yogurt
- Splash of water
- Ice cubes

Method:

1. Blend the strawberries, kiwi, yogurt, and water until smooth.
2. Blend in ice cubes for a refreshing and vitamin-rich smoothie.

Nutritional Info:

Calories: 130 / Protein: 3g / Fiber: 4g / Potassium: 180mg / Phosphorus: 40mg / Sodium: 30mg

Mango Lime Twist

Prep Time: 5 minutes
Blending Time: 2 minutes
Ingredients:

- 1/2 cup mango chunks
- Juice of 1 lime
- 1/2 cup low-potassium coconut water
- Ice cubes

Method:

1. Blend the mango, lime juice, and coconut water until smooth.
2. Add ice cubes and combine to create a tropical and zesty treat.

Nutritional Info:

Calories: 110 / Protein: 1g / Fiber: 3g / Potassium: 130mg / Phosphorus: 30mg / Sodium: 20mg

Spinach Blueberry Booster

Prep Time: 5 minutes
Blending Time: 2 minutes
Ingredients:

*   Handful of fresh spinach leaves
*   1/2 cup blueberries
*   1/2 banana
*   1/2 cup low-sodium almond milk
*   Ice cubes

Method:

1. Blend spinach, blueberries, banana, and almond milk until thoroughly incorporated.
2. Add ice cubes and combine to make a nutrient-dense green smoothie.

Nutritional Info:

Calories: 110 / Protein: 2g / Fiber: 4g / Potassium: 210mg / Phosphorus: 40mg / Sodium: 70mg

Cherry Almond Delight

Prep Time: 5 minutes
Blending Time: 2 minutes
Ingredients:

- 1/2 cup cherries, pitted
- 1 tablespoon almond butter (low phosphorus)
- 1/2 cup low-sodium almond milk
- Ice cubes

Method:

1. Blend the cherries, almond butter, and almond milk until creamy.
2. Add ice cubes and combine to make a wonderfully nutty smoothie.

Nutritional Info:
Calories: 160 / Protein: 4g / Fiber: 3g / Potassium: 180mg / Phosphorus: 60mg / Sodium: 60mg

Papaya Orange Sunrise

Prep Time: 5 minutes
Blending Time: 2 minutes
Ingredients:

- 1/2 cup papaya chunks
- Juice of 1 orange
- 1/2 cup low-potassium coconut water
- Ice cubes

Method:

1. Blend the papaya, orange juice, and coconut water until smooth.
2. Add ice cubes and combine to create a tropical dawn in a glass.

Nutritional Info:

Calories: 120 / Protein: 1g / Fiber: 2g / Potassium: 110mg / Phosphorus: 30mg / Sodium: 20mg

Vanilla Pear Dream

Prep Time: 5 minutes
Blending Time: 2 minutes
Ingredients:

- 1/2 pear, sliced
- 1/2 teaspoon vanilla extract
- 1/2 cup low-sodium almond milk
- Ice cubes

Method:

1. Blend the pear pieces, vanilla extract, and almond milk until smooth.
2. Add ice cubes and combine to make a sweet and pleasant smoothie.

Nutritional Info:

Calories: 130 / Protein: 2g / Fiber: 4g / Potassium: 160mg / Phosphorus: 40mg / Sodium: 70mg

Snack Recipes

Roasted Chickpeas

Prep Time: 5 minutes
Cooking Time: 30 minutes
Ingredients:

- 1 can (15 ounces) chickpeas, drained and rinsed
- Olive oil (low sodium)
- Garlic powder, cumin, paprika
- Salt to taste

Method:

1. Mix chickpeas with olive oil and spices.
2. Roast in the oven until crisp.

Nutritional Info:

Calories: 150 / Protein: 6g / Fiber: 5g / Potassium: 180mg /
Phosphorus: 100mg / Sodium: 70mg

Vegetable Sticks with Hummus

Prep Time: 10 minutes
Cooking Time: 0 minutes
Ingredients:

- Carrot, cucumber, and celery sticks
- Low-sodium hummus

Method:

1. Cut the vegetables into sticks.
2. Serve with a side of hummus to dip.

Nutritional Info:
Calories: 80 / Protein: 3g / Fiber: 4g / Potassium: 150mg /
Phosphorus: 60mg / Sodium: 50mg

Greek Yogurt Parfait

Prep Time: 5 minutes
Cooking Time: 0 minutes
Ingredients:

- 1/2 cup low-fat Greek yogurt
- Berries (strawberries, blueberries)
- Granola (low phosphorus)
- 1 teaspoon honey (optional)

Method:

1. Combine yogurt, berries, and granola.
2. Drizzle with honey if preferred.

Nutritional Info:
Calories: 180 / Protein: 10g / Fiber: 3g / Potassium: 200mg
/ Phosphorus: 70mg / Sodium: 50mg

Apple and Almond Butter Slices

Prep Time: 5 minutes
Cooking Time: 0 minutes
Ingredients:

- Apple slices
- Almond butter (low phosphorus)

Method:
1. Spread almond butter on apple slices.

Nutritional Info:
Calories: 120 / Protein: 3g / Fiber: 4g / Potassium: 180mg / Phosphorus: 50mg / Sodium: 10mg

Edamame Snack

Prep Time: 5 minutes
Cooking Time: 5 minutes
Ingredients:
- Edamame, steamed
- Sea salt

Method:
1. Steam edamame and sprinkle with sea salt.

Nutritional Info:
Calories: 100 / Protein: 9g / Fiber: 4g / Potassium: 150mg / Phosphorus: 90mg / Sodium: 5mg

Rice Cake with Avocado

Prep Time: 5 minutes
Cooking Time: 0 minutes
Ingredients:
- Low-sodium rice cake
- Avocado slices
- Sprinkle of sesame seeds

Method:

2. Cut avocado slices and place them on top of the rice cake.
3. Sprinkle with sesame seeds.

Nutritional Info:

Calories: 130 / Protein: 2g / Fiber: 3g / Potassium: 220mg / Phosphorus: 40mg / Sodium: 20mg

Cottage Cheese and Pineapple Cups

Prep Time: 5 minutes
Cooking Time: 0 minutes
Ingredients:

- Low-sodium cottage cheese
- Pineapple chunks

Method:

1. Fill small cups with cottage cheese and top with pineapple.

Nutritional Info:

Calories: 120 / Protein: 12g / Fiber: 1g / Potassium: 150mg / Phosphorus: 100mg / Sodium: 70mg

Trail Mix with Nuts and Seeds

Prep Time: 5 minutes
Cooking Time: 0 minutes
Ingredients:
- Mixed nuts (almonds, walnuts)
- Pumpkin seeds
- Dried cranberries (unsweetened)

Method:
1. Mix nuts, seeds, and cranberries together.

Nutritional Info:
Calories: 160 / Protein: 5g / Fiber: 3g / Potassium: 170mg /
Phosphorus: 90mg / Sodium: 5mg

Kale Chips

Prep Time: 10 minutes
Cooking Time: 15 minutes
Ingredients:
- Fresh kale leaves
- Olive oil (low sodium)
- Nutritional yeast
- Sea salt

Method:
1. Massage the kale with olive oil, nutritional yeast, and salt.
2. Bake till crisp.

Nutritional Info:
Calories: 70 / Protein: 3g / Fiber: 2g / Potassium: 240mg / Phosphorus: 60mg / Sodium: 40mg

Chia Pudding with Berries

Prep Time: 5 minutes
Chilling Time: 2 hours
Ingredients:
- 2 tablespoons chia seeds
- 1/2 cup low-potassium almond milk
- Mixed berries

Method:
1. Combine chia seeds and almond milk; refrigerate until pudding-like.
2. Before serving, top with a combination of berries.

Nutritional Info:
Calories: 120 / Protein: 4g / Fiber: 6g / Potassium: 90mg / Phosphorus: 40mg / Sodium: 10mg

28-Day Meal Plan

Feel free to customize this simplified meal plan according to individual preferences and dietary needs. Remember to stay hydrated and enjoy the journey to a healthier lifestyle!

WEEK 1 MEAL PLAN

Dates
____

	BREAKFAST	LUNCH	DINNER	SNACKS
MON	Berry Blast Smoothie	Greek Yogurt Parfait	Baked Lemon Herb Chicken / Quinoa Salad	Roasted Chickpeas
TUE	Apple and Almond Butter Slices	Vegetable Sticks with Hummus	Tofu and Vegetable Stir-Fry / Brown Rice	Edamame Snack
WED	Mango Lime Twist	Rice Cake with Avocado	Grilled Salmon / Sweet Potato Wedges	Greek Yogurt Parfait
THU	Cucumber Mint Refresher	Roasted Chickpeas	Chicken and Vegetable Skewers / Quinoa	Apple and Almond Butter Slices
FRI	Strawberry Kiwi Delight	Trail Mix with Nuts and Seeds	Eggplant and Tomato Bake / Cauliflower Rice	Cottage Cheese and Pineapple Cups
SAT	Avocado Banana Bliss	Greek Salad with Feta	Lentil Soup / Whole Wheat Roll	Berry Blast Smoothie
SUN	Vanilla Pear Dream	Chia Pudding with Berries	Shrimp Stir-Fry / Steamed Broccoli	Kale Chips

Shopping list

WEEK 2 MEAL PLAN

Dates

____

	BREAKFAST	LUNCH	DINNER	SNACKS
MON	Pineapple Ginger Zing	Apple and Almond Butter Slices	Grilled Chicken Salad / Quinoa	Roasted Chickpeas
TUE	Berry Blast Smoothie	Rice Cake with Avocado	Baked Cod with Herbs / Asparagus	Edamame Snack
WED	Chia Pudding with Berries	Greek Yogurt Parfait	Tofu and Vegetable Stir-Fry / Brown Rice	Trail Mix with Nuts and Seeds
THU	Vanilla Pear Dream	Vegetable Sticks with Hummus	Chicken and Broccoli Casserole / Quinoa	Cottage Cheese and Pineapple Cups
FRI	Mango Lime Twist	Roasted Chickpeas	Lentil Curry / Basmati Rice	Greek Yogurt Parfait
SAT	Avocado Banana Bliss	Kale Chips	Baked Lemon Herb Chicken / Roasted Sweet Potatoes	Apple and Almond Butter Slices
SUN	Cucumber Mint Refresher	Trail Mix with Nuts and Seeds	Grilled Salmon / Steamed Broccoli	Berry Blast Smoothie

Shopping list

WEEK 3 MEAL PLAN

Dates

____

	BREAKFAST	LUNCH	DINNER	SNACKS
MON	Vanilla Pear Dream	Chia Pudding with Berries	Eggplant and Tomato Bake / Quinoa	Roasted Chickpeas
TUE	Berry Blast Smoothie	Greek Yogurt Parfait	Shrimp Stir-Fry / Brown Rice	Edamame Snack
WED	Apple and Almond Butter Slices	Vegetable Sticks with Hummus	Baked Cod with Herbs / Asparagus	Trail Mix with Nuts and Seeds
THU	Cucumber Mint Refresher	Rice Cake with Avocado	Grilled Chicken Salad / Cauliflower Rice	Cottage Cheese and Pineapple Cups
FRI	Strawberry Kiwi Delight	Trail Mix with Nuts and Seeds	Lentil Soup / Whole Wheat Roll	Greek Yogurt Parfait
SAT	Avocado Banana Bliss	Kale Chips	Tofu and Vegetable Stir-Fry / Quinoa	Apple and Almond Butter Slices
SUN	Mango Lime Twist	Chia Pudding with Berries	Baked Lemon Herb Chicken / Roasted Sweet Potatoes	Roasted Chickpeas

Shopping list

WEEK 4 MEAL PLAN

Dates
____

	BREAKFAST	LUNCH	DINNER	SNACKS
MON	Pineapple Ginger Zing	Greek Yogurt Parfait	Lentil Curry / Basmati Rice	Edamame Snack
TUE	Berry Blast Smoothie	Rice Cake with Avocado	Shrimp Stir-Fry / Brown Rice	Trail Mix with Nuts and Seeds
WED	Chia Pudding with Berries	Vegetable Sticks with Hummus	Chicken and Vegetable Skewers / Quinoa	Cottage Cheese and Pineapple Cups
THU	Vanilla Pear Dream	Roasted Chickpeas	Grilled Salmon / Steamed Broccoli	Greek Yogurt Parfait
FRI	Mango Lime Twist	Trail Mix with Nuts and Seeds	Eggplant and Tomato Bake / Cauliflower Rice	Apple and Almond Butter Slices
SAT	Avocado Banana Bliss	Kale Chips	Baked Cod with Herbs / Asparagus	Roasted Chickpeas
SUN	Cucumber Mint Refresher	Greek Yogurt Parfait	Tofu and Vegetable Stir-Fry / Brown Rice	Berry Blast Smoothie

Shopping list

CONCLUSION

In the last pages of "Kidney Disease Cookbook for Stage 3," we arrive not only at the finish, but also at the beginning of a new journey—one full of health, vigor, and a profound appreciation of nutrition's transformative potential. As we say goodbye to the pages that have taken us through healthy recipes, enlightening information, and experiences of others who have discovered new hope, it's important to consider the significant impact that a conscious and intentional diet can have on our lives.

The trip we've taken together goes beyond what a cookbook can offer. It demonstrates the persistence of the human spirit and the body's extraordinary ability to heal when given the correct tools. Through the lens of managing Stage 3 Renal Disease, we've seen triumphant stories, accepted the wisdom of a nephrologist-approved low sodium, low potassium, and low phosphorus diet, and experienced the joy of purposefully nourishing our bodies.

For many people, this book is more than simply a cookbook; it's a lifeline—a guide to negotiating the challenges of renal health with elegance, flavor, and a dash of culinary talent. It's a guide on the way to regaining control of our health, demonstrating that every meal is an opportunity for healing, growth, and celebration of life.

As you close this book, I encourage you to use the ideas taught within its pages. Let these dishes serve as the cornerstone for a healthy, long-lasting lifestyle. Enjoy each bite with the awareness that you are making decisions that nourish not only your body but also your spirit, demonstrating your dedication to a healthy, thriving existence.

Remember that the path to optimal health is not without hurdles. There may be times when the journey appears steep, but let this cookbook serve as a compass, directing you back to the comforting embrace of healthful, kidney-friendly cuisine. Embrace the delight of kitchen experimentation, infusing each dish with your own personality, and enjoy the flavors that dance on your taste receptors.

As we part ways within the pages of this book, remember that the knowledge you've gained is a gift, and you have the potential to alter your health. The road does not end here; it continues with every grocery trip, mindful meal preparation, and conscious daily decisions.

I am deeply grateful to you for prioritizing your health and for your unwavering commitment to treating Stage 3 Renal Disease with grace and persistence. It has been an honor to be a part of your path, and I genuinely hope that this book has provided inspiration, advice, and empowerment.

In conclusion, I ask you to reflect on the good adjustments you've made, the newfound vitality you've discovered, and the delectable flavors that have adorned your plate. Your experience with this cookbook is invaluable, and I would be happy if you could share your insights with others who could benefit from this transforming trip.

If you found this book to be a great resource, I would appreciate it if you could leave a review and rating on Amazon, Goodreads, or any other site where you purchased it. Your review has the potential to reach others looking for advice on their kidney health journey, providing them with a glimpse into the transformational potential contained within these pages.

Your comment is more than just a review; it is a beacon of hope for someone looking for answers, and it serves as an inspiration for people dealing with renal disease. Let us work together to build a supportive community by sharing our experiences and thoughts to inspire and help others on their journey to optimal health.

Thank you again for letting me be a part of your journey. May your days be full with health, joy, and the delightful pleasure of indulging in the bright tastes of a well-nourished existence.

RECIPE JOURNAL

Recipe:

Prep Time: CookingTime: No. Of Serves:

Ingredients

Cooking Directions

Notes

Recipe:

Prep Time: CookingTime: No. Of Serves:

Ingredients

Cooking Directions

Notes

Recipe:

Prep Time: **CookingTime:**   **No. Of Serves:**

Ingredients

Cooking Directions

Notes

Recipe:

Prep Time: **CookingTime:**   **No. Of Serves:**

Ingredients

Cooking Directions

Notes

Recipe:

Prep Time: **CookingTime:**   **No. Of Serves:**

Ingredients

Cooking Directions

Notes

Recipe:

Prep Time: **CookingTime:**   **No. Of Serves:**

Ingredients

Cooking Directions

Notes

Recipe:

Prep Time: **CookingTime:**   **No. Of Serves:**

Ingredients

Cooking Directions

Notes

Recipe:
Prep Time: CookingTime: No. Of Serves:
Ingredients
Cooking Directions
Notes

Recipe:
Prep Time: CookingTime: No. Of Serves:
Ingredients
Cooking Directions
Notes

Recipe:
Prep Time: CookingTime: No. Of Serves:
Ingredients
Cooking Directions
Notes

Recipe:

Prep Time: **Cooking Time:**   **No. Of Serves:**

Ingredients

Cooking Directions

Notes

Recipe:

Prep Time: CookingTime: No. Of Serves:

Ingredients

Cooking Directions

Notes

Recipe:

Prep Time: CookingTime: No. Of Serves:

Ingredients

Cooking Directions

Notes

Recipe:

Prep Time: **Cooking Time:**   **No. Of Serves:**

Ingredients

Cooking Directions

Notes

Recipe:

Prep Time: CookingTime: No. Of Serves:

Ingredients

Cooking Directions

Notes

Recipe:

Prep Time: **CookingTime:**   **No. Of Serves:**

Ingredients

Cooking Directions

Notes

Recipe:

Prep Time: **CookingTime:**   **No. Of Serves:**

Ingredients

Cooking Directions

Notes

Recipe: [   ]

Prep Time: **CookingTime:**   **No. Of Serves:**

Ingredients

Cooking Directions

Notes

Recipe: [   ]

Prep Time: CookingTime: No. Of Serves:

Ingredients

Cooking Directions

Notes

Recipe:

Prep Time: **CookingTime:**   **No. Of Serves:**

Ingredients

Cooking Directions

Notes

Recipe:

Prep Time: **CookingTime:**   **No. Of Serves:**

Ingredients

Cooking Directions

Notes

Recipe:

Prep Time: **CookingTime:**   **No. Of Serves:**

Ingredients

Cooking Directions

Notes

Recipe:

Prep Time: **CookingTime:**   **No. Of Serves:**

Ingredients

Cooking Directions

Notes

Recipe:

Prep Time: **CookingTime:**   **No. Of Serves:**

Ingredients

Cooking Directions

Notes

Recipe:
Prep Time: CookingTime: No. Of Serves:
Ingredients
Cooking Directions
Notes

Recipe:
Prep Time: CookingTime: No. Of Serves:
Ingredients
Cooking Directions
Notes

Recipe:

Prep Time: **CookingTime:**   **No. Of Serves:**

Ingredients

Cooking Directions

Notes